DIET PROOF
YOUR LIFE

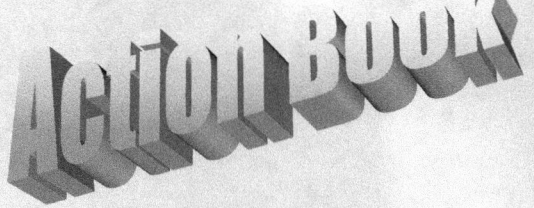

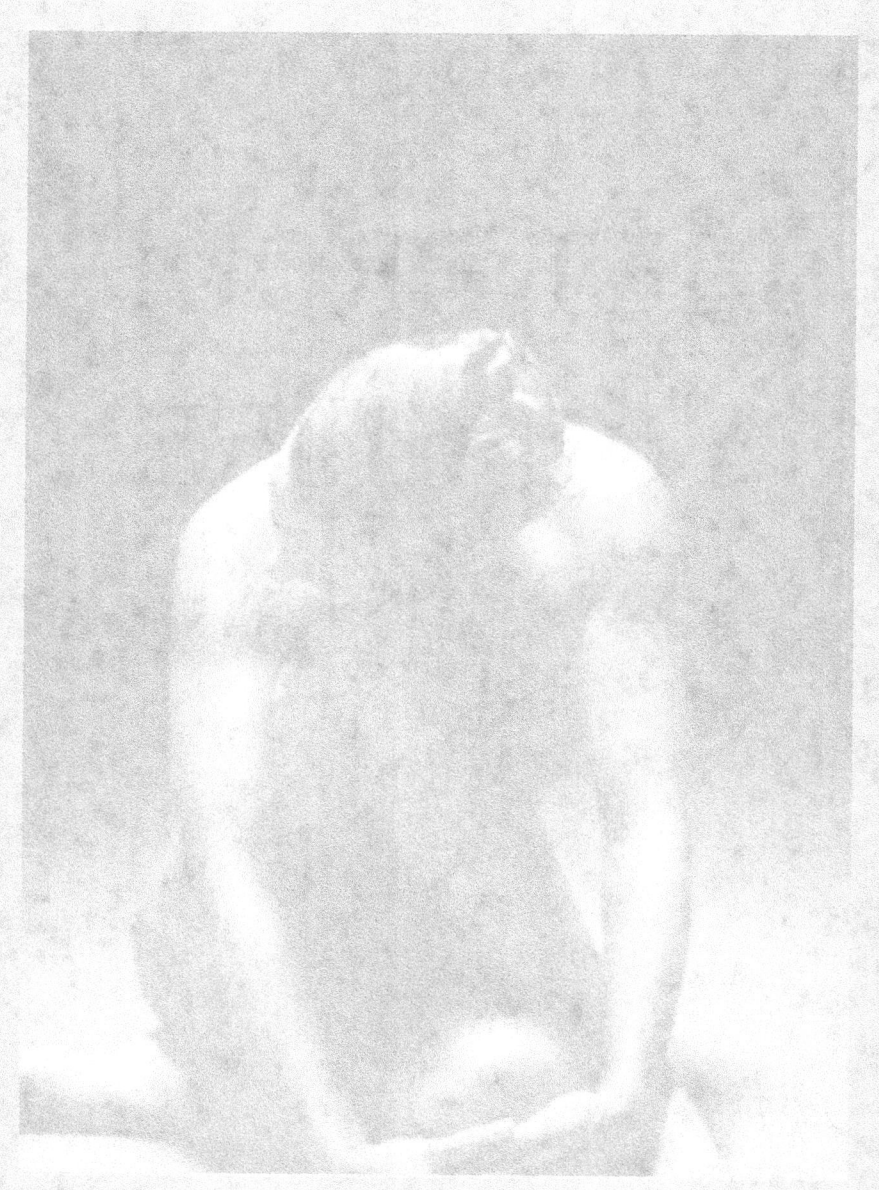

DIET PROOF YOUR LIFE

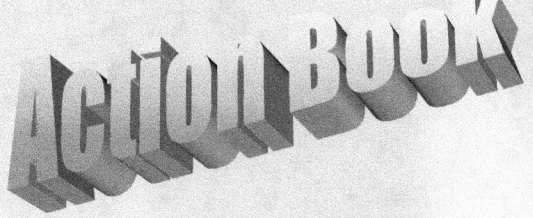

Yael Eylat-Tanaka

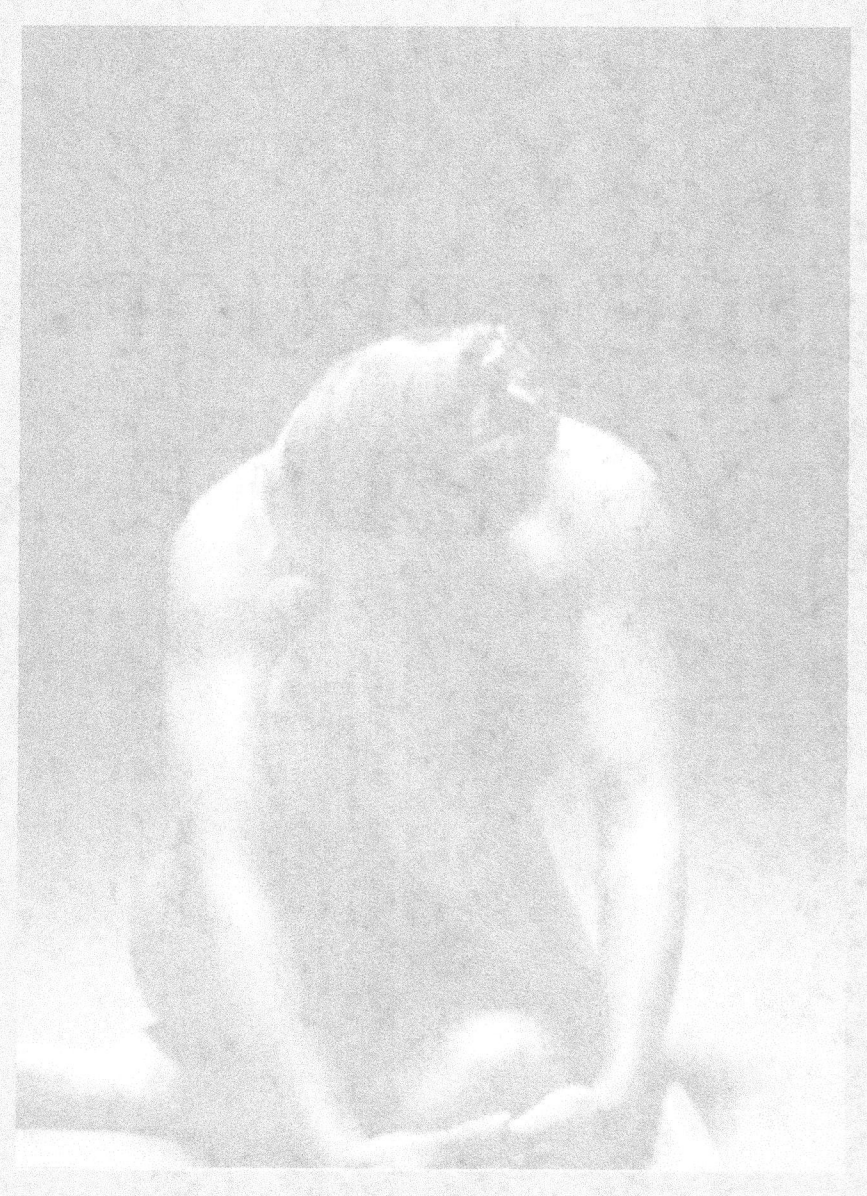

Copyright

Disclaimer

This book is meant to inspire you to take a journey of self-discovery, and thus attain a measure of serenity and self-acceptance. Nothing in this book is intended as a substitute for medical advice. Please consult your own medical professional for any personal medical issues or specific recommendations.

Other Books by the Author

Diet Proof Your Life: The Seven Essential Secrets of Success
Common Bits of Life
Dreams – Poetry of the Mind
Lake of Silence
The Book of Values
Publish Your Book Using CreateSpace
Publish Your Book on Kindle
Publish Your Book With NOOK Press
Publish Your eBook on Smashwords
Publish Your eBook on BookTango
SCREAMS! Three short stories of terror
Revenge of the Cat Woman

Acknowledgments

After publishing Diet Proof Your Life: The Seven Essential Secrets of Success, several people commented that a workbook might be useful as a tool to practice those secrets. It is therefore with great pleasure that I have produced this book. Thank you to all who contributed! I specifically acknowledge my friend and colleague, Dr. John E. Christ, for his advice on the physiology of dieting. His encouragement served to channel my writing. My deep gratitude goes to Frankie Nickerson for holding my feet to the fire in discussing the values that are the backbone of this book, and my sister, Dr. Dina Eisen, who so deeply believes in the tenets put forth in my book. Her vision and calm demeanor exemplify optimal health and well-being of body and spirit.

Contents

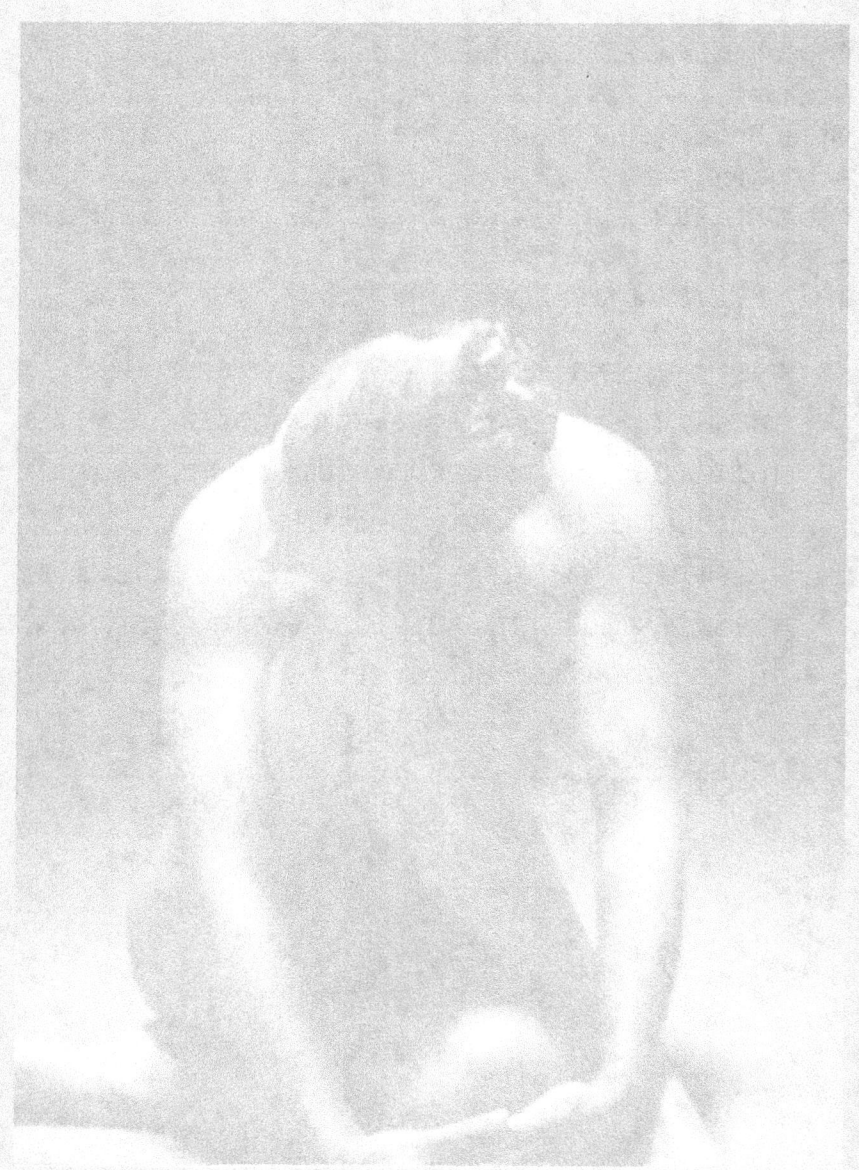

INTRODUCTION

This Action Book is yours – exclusively. It is a private repository of your thoughts, secrets, aspirations and successes. The more honestly you reveal yourself in these pages, the more benefit you will receive. It is your journal. It is your gift to yourself.

I initially wrote *Diet Proof Your Life* as a journal. I wanted to examine what was at the core of my overweight; what lay beneath the depression and discontent I experienced, even though at first I could not acknowledge my depression; more specifically, I could not associate my depression with my weight. Indeed, as I continued my journey, I came to realize what was obvious all along: My weight was a mere reflection of how I felt; my inner being needed to be addressed before my weight would reflect the real "me." Even more to the point, my weight was not the issue at all – it was my style of dealing with life: my eating style.

It was a circuitous journey. Which came first – the weight or the underlying misery? Could it be that my eating and food choices were so out of kilter as to cause of my misery? A process of personal examination ensued, and the book *Diet Proof Your Life* was born. I became convinced that I was not alone in my struggle, and that my struggle was universal, and was not being addressed. While the media focused on weight loss or weight control, there was never any talk of other integral issues that contributed to the epidemic of overweight. It therefore became my mission to examine those principles, and bring to the fore a new paradigm.

The journey was elucidating. Interestingly, as soon as I resolved to take hold of my problem, I surrendered. From

1

that point on, I was no longer white-knuckling my way through yet another deprivation diet. I no longer counted the days until I could eat "normally" again. I changed my focus from losing weight to recovery. I resolved to discover what recovery meant for me, what was it I needed to recover from. The most immediate answer was that I needed to recover from using food to self-medicate. Yes, that was a big one.

When I realized that I used food as a drug, a whole world opened up for me to unravel: Me, on drugs?? I had never taken drugs in my life! I read everything I could on how food functioned, what effect certain foods had on the body and the brain, how certain foods were addictive, and why I craved more and more, even when full. Why was I not sated when others could eat a reasonable amount and get up from the table?

My quest took me in unexpected directions, on foreign soil and surprising revelations. Seemingly unrelated factors united to produce a picture that solidified in my mind. I began to understand.

Learn to challenge your own story. Reframe the events in your life. Do not compare yourself to others; do not torment yourself by what might have been. Be wise in accepting criticism – if it is valid, acknowledge it and move on; if not, reject it. Let go of expectations that others behave as you want them to. Focus on yourself, because you are the only one you can control.

This journey is yours. Enjoy it. Enjoy where you are at this moment. Revel in the process of discovery. Practice mindful eating. Each time you complete an assignment, celebrate that. As you are reading and writing your assignments, enjoy the process of looking within. All life is a continuum, a road on which you live a day at a time, with landmarks along the way. Enjoy them all.

The subtitle of the book is *The Seven Essential Secrets of Success,* but in fact, there are many other secrets that play a vital role in any endeavor, be it taking care of your physical body, or raising happy children. These "secrets" are principles that are integral to a life well lived, such as forbearance, wisdom, courage, tenacity, responsibility and humility. I invite you to read *The Book of Values*, where I discuss 140 human values (Amazon.com). Cherish and nurture your relationships, and avoid toxic ones.

Balance work with play. Balance implies doing what is necessary to support your life, and then resting and experiencing a sense of peace and relaxation. Protect your psychic energy.

Above all, have fun. Let yourself go; tell your deepest secrets; explore your fears; express your angers and resentments within these pages, then let them go. These pages are meant to encourage you as you discover your inner soul.

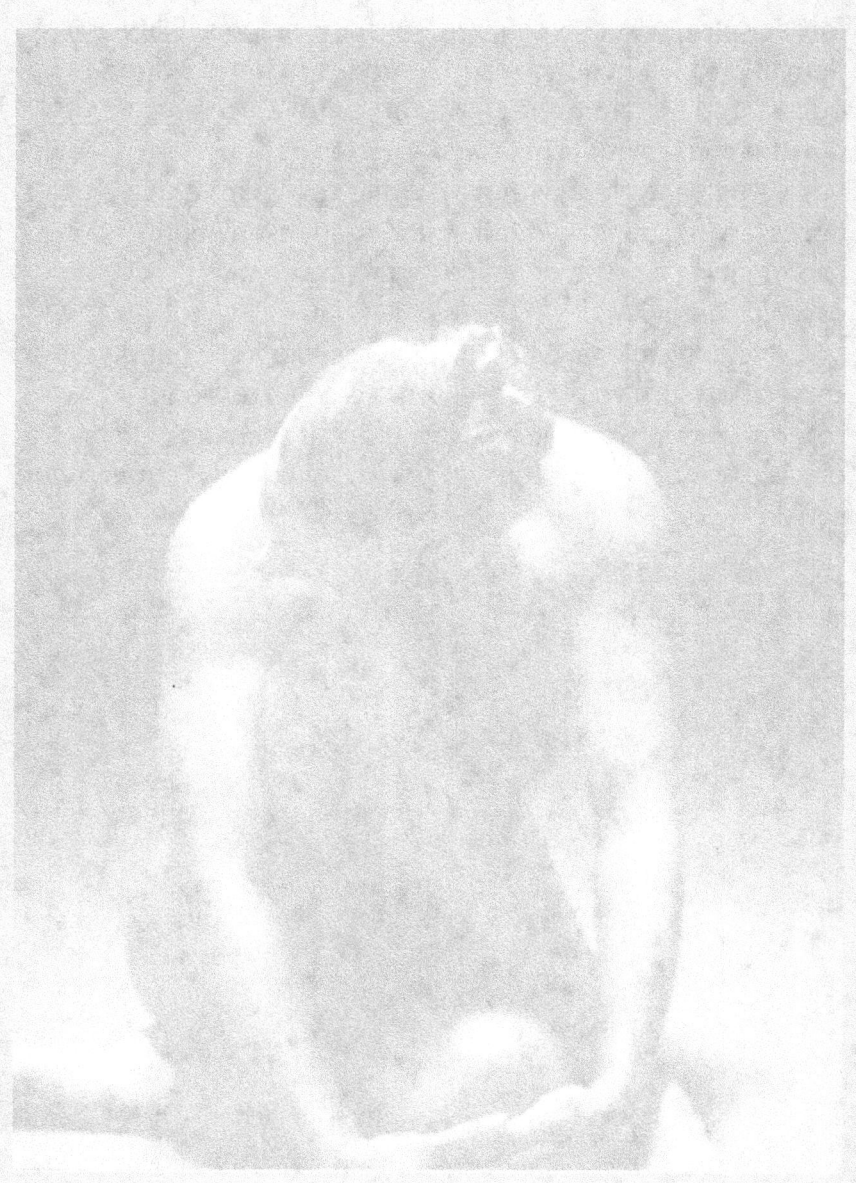

THE 7 ESSENTIAL

SECRETS OF SUCCESS

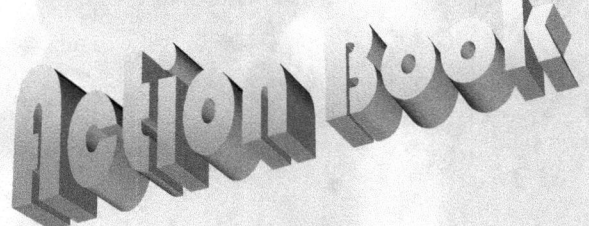

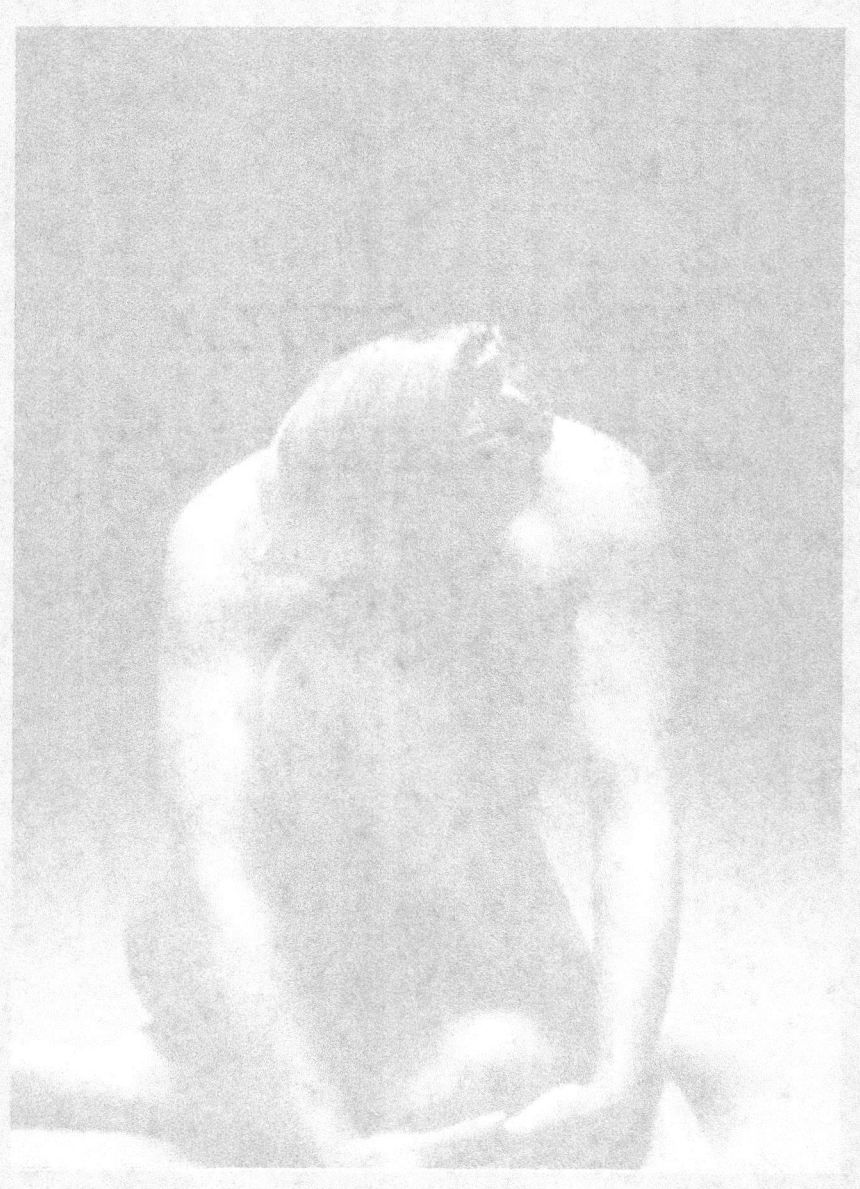

THE FIRST SECRET:
EXERCISE

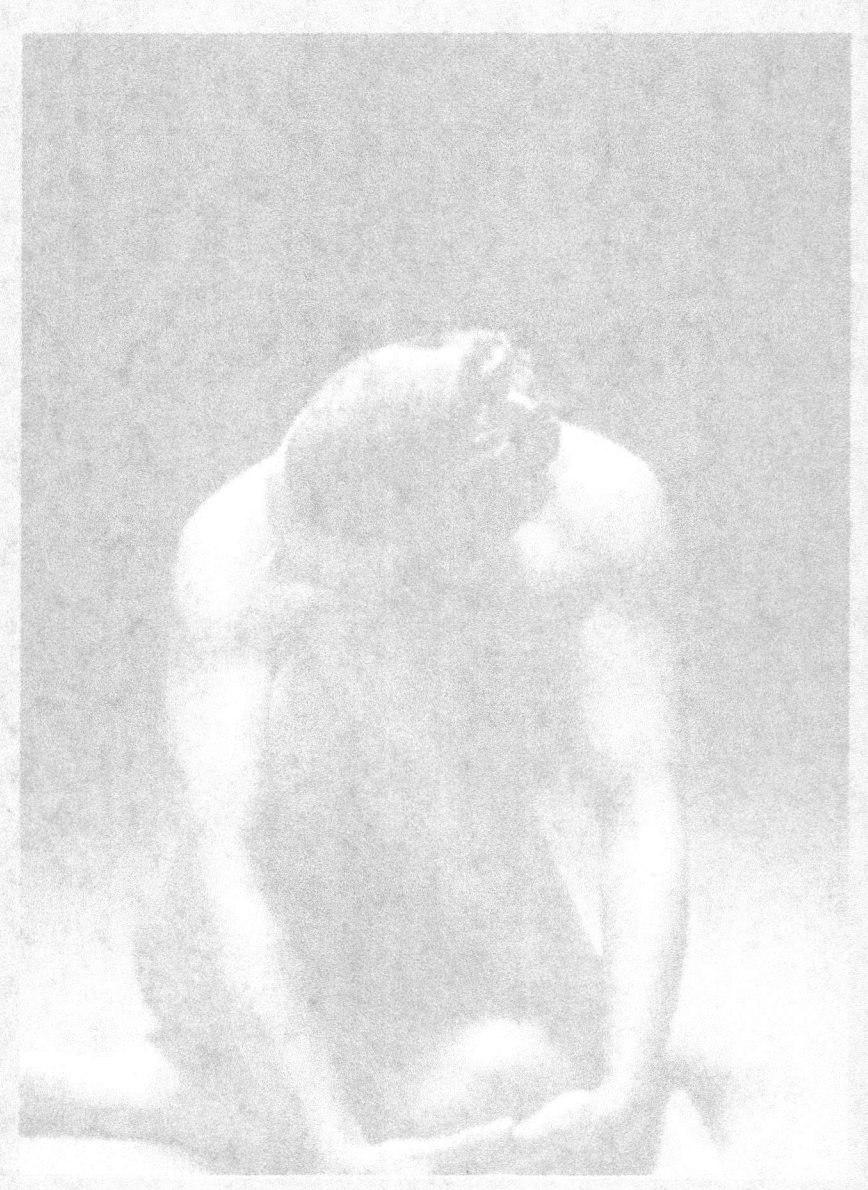

The benefits of regular exercise are almost too numerous to recite. They range from burning calories to revving up your metabolism; producing endorphins to forestalling infirmity in old age; protecting against many kinds of cancer to reducing your appetite; improving your cognition by oxygenating the brain to improving your sexual response and sleep.

Do you exercise regularly? If not, why not?

What kind of exercise to you engage in?
- Aerobic – running, swimming, biking, dancing, walking
- Non-aerobic – weight lifting
- Both?

If you do not exercise, or get only minimal exercise, why?
- No interest
- No time
- No place

How would you design your perfect exercise routine?
- Time
- Place

How long do you typically exercise?

Do you feel that's enough? If not, why not?

What would make your exercise session more productive or more beneficial?

What would make exercise more enjoyable?

Exercise is beneficial for its own sake, but many people exercise to get a specific result. What result are you seeking?
- I want to lose weight
- I want to tone my body
- I want to spend time with my friends

Do you tend to give up after only a few days if you do not get the desired results? Do you feel discouraged?

How do you feel after you exercise?
- Exhausted
- Exhilarated
- Uplifted
- Terrible!
- I'm never gonna do that again!

If you had a magic wand and could wave it over your exercise routine, what would it look like?

After exercising vigorously, do you enjoy relaxing and winding down?

- Yes
- No
- Why?

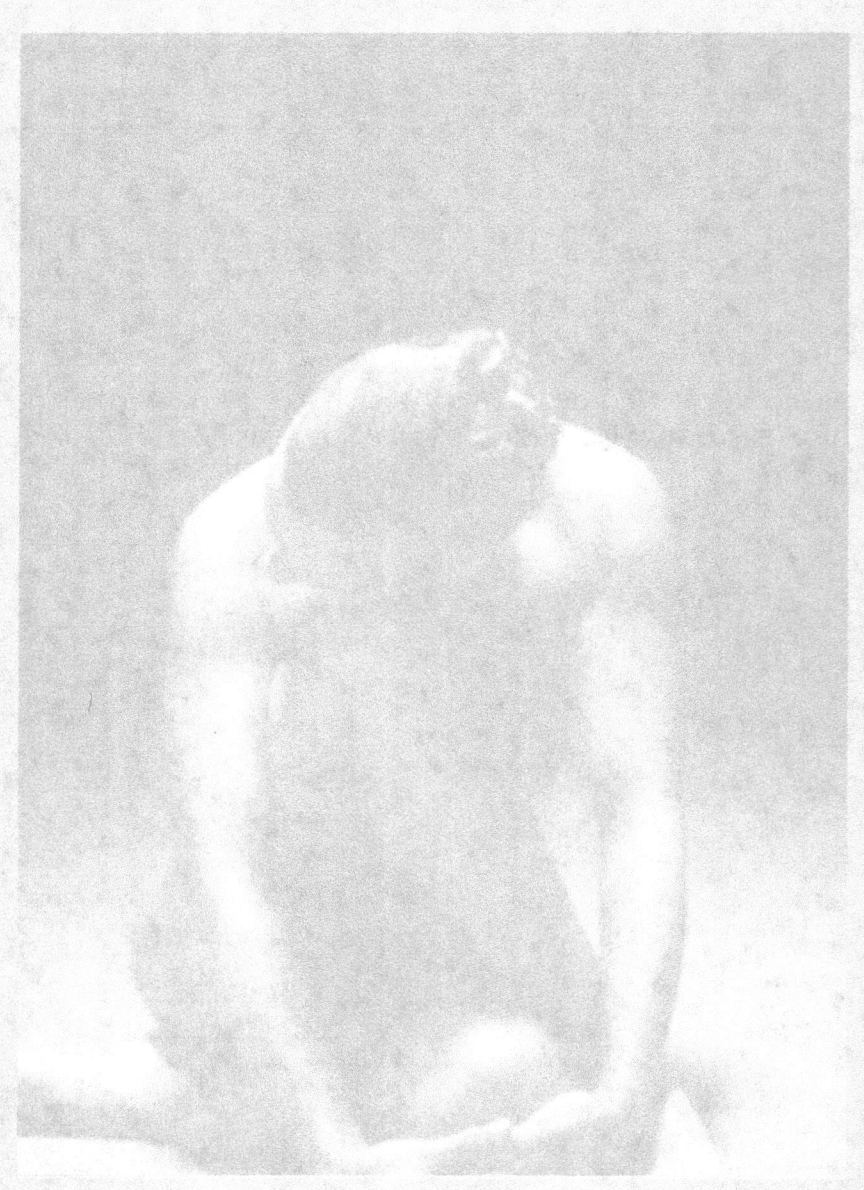

THE SECOND SECRET:
AVOID TRIGGER FOODS

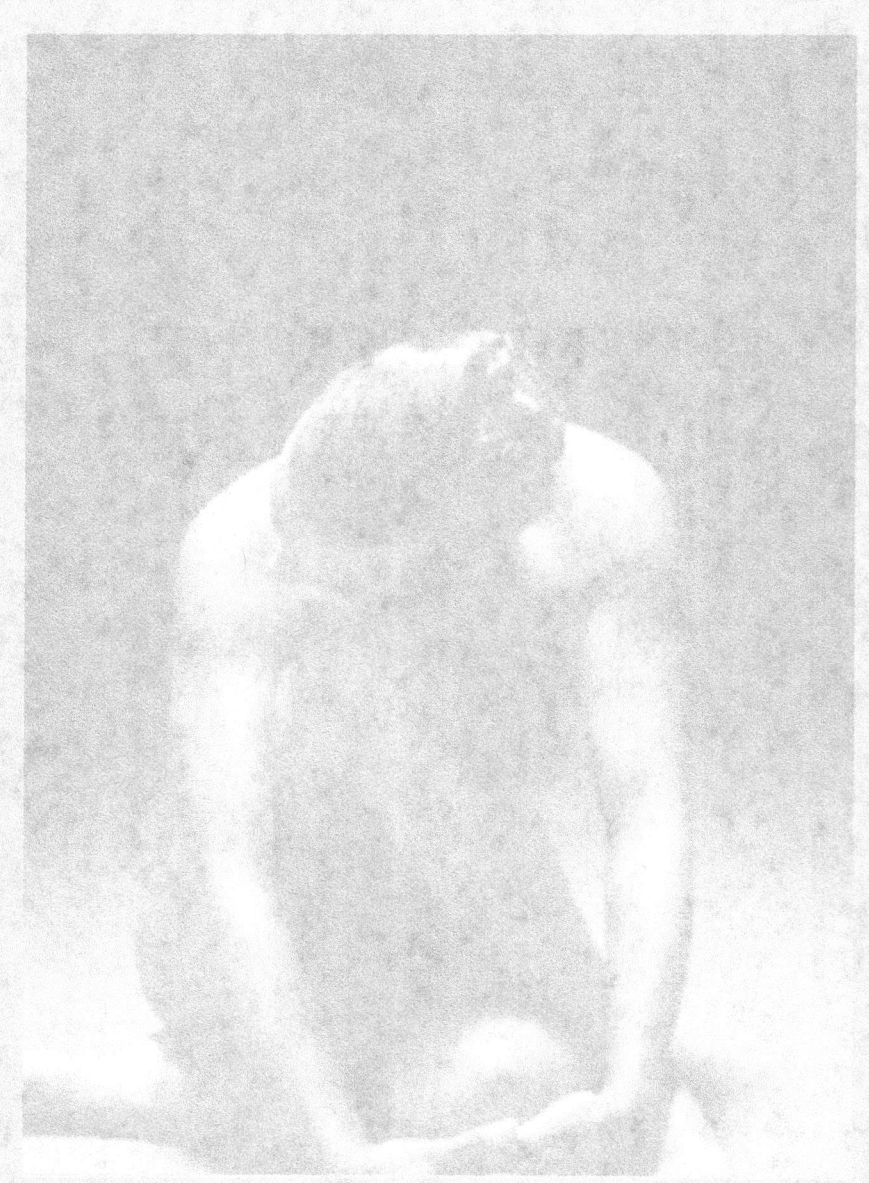

A "trigger food" is any food that you cannot consume in reasonable quantities. Reasonable is relative, of course. To be a trigger, a food item may be the cause for a binge, either immediately or at a later time, or may be an item that you cannot control. For example, one of my trigger foods is roasted nuts. Even though I know that nuts are healthy, the usual recommendation is a handful. I am not able to take a handful of roasted nuts and leave the rest. If I get started, the bottom of the jar is close at hand. I therefore prefer to not start.

On a scale from 1-10, how problematic are trigger foods in your eating self-control?

_____

List some or all your particular trigger foods:

_____

_____

_____

_____

_____

_____

_____

_____

_____

_____

How do you behave or respond to a trigger food?

_____

_____

Are you able to control yourself, or are you compelled to eat it?

Do you eat trigger foods alone? Do you hide wrappers from others?

How do you feel after you have binged on a trigger food? Be as specific and thorough as you can – this is your private workbook.

- I feel dirty
- I feel depressed
- I hate myself

This chapter is about clarifying some of your trigger foods; but "trigger situations" are also quite relevant to your overall well-being.

How do you respond to loneliness? Upset? Jealousy? Does stress cause you to overeat? Describe areas of stress in your life:

- My family
- My job
- My friends

THE THIRD SECRET: REDISCOVER YOUR FAVORITE FOODS

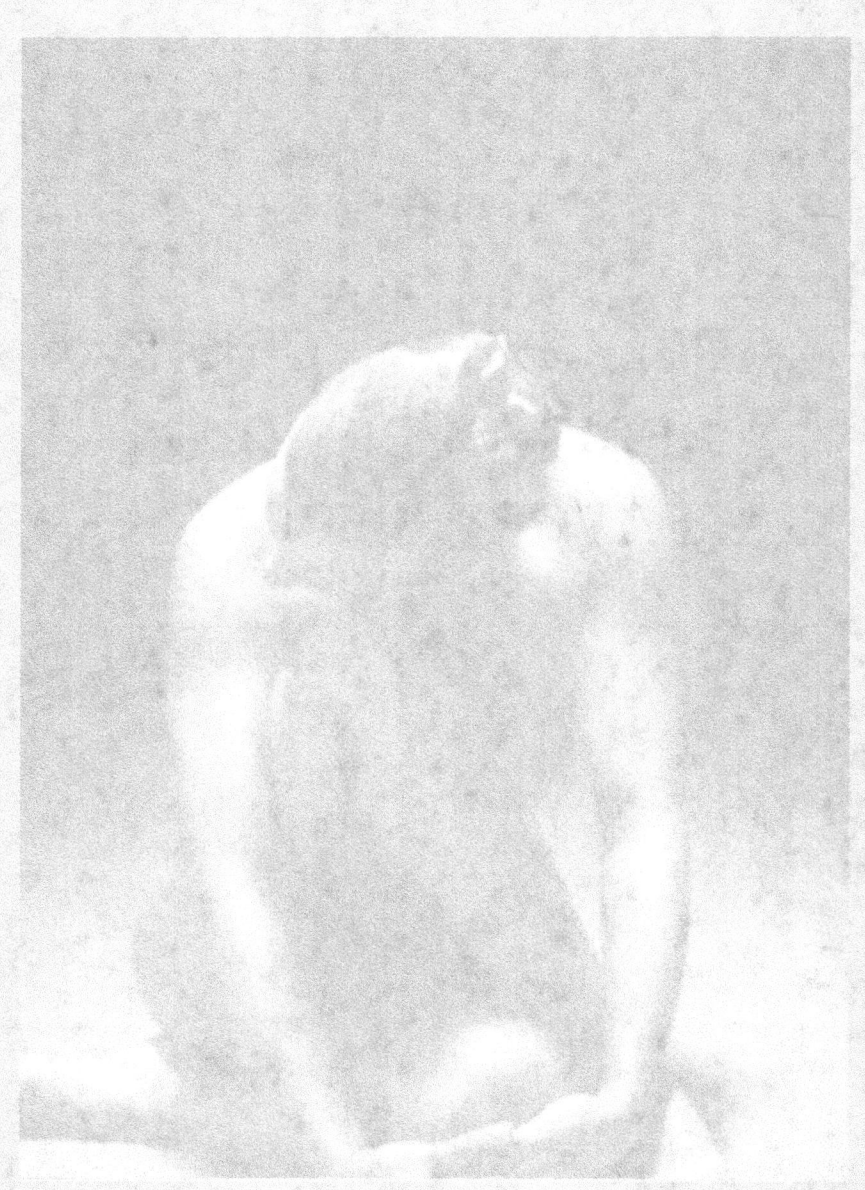

When we overeat, especially trigger foods, processed foods, celebratory foods, we tend to keep on eating those foods out of habit. These habits – grabbing something quick at a fast food restaurant, or passing by the drive-through window for a milkshake, or buying a bag of chips at the local store – take a hold of us and we forget that we have other foods we love, foods that are as wholesome as they are delicious. For example, one of my favorite dishes from childhood is *bamias*, a stew of okra, corn and tomatoes that my grandmother made. I recently reminded a friend of *bamias*, and we both began salivating at the memory; and yet, I rarely prepare it. Why? Habit. Other favorite foods are carrot salads dressed with sugar and lemon - nothing is so refreshing on a hot summer day. I also love roasted eggplant and baked tomatoes. So why don't I indulge more often? Habit.

Allow your mind to float back to your childhood. Recall some favorite foods you had then that were not processed. Name some here.

- What food have you not eaten in a long time?
- What was your favorite food as a child?
- Was/is your favorite food processed or natural?

Are these foods readily available now? Do you know where to find them? Could you prepare them yourself?

If they require a special recipe, can you find it from family members? From the internet?

Processed foods are those that do not occur naturally, such as fruits or vegetables. If a food product has a list of ingredients, it is processed. For optimum health, physical and mental, you should endeavor to consume the least processed food available, such as traditional oatmeal (Ingredients: 100% oats), or any food found in nature. An apple is natural in its natural state; packaged cereal is not.

- Do you ever read the ingredient list? If not, why not?
- Do you enjoy natural, unprocessed foods?
- Do you tend to crave fatty foods?
- What are your go-to foods when you are upset?

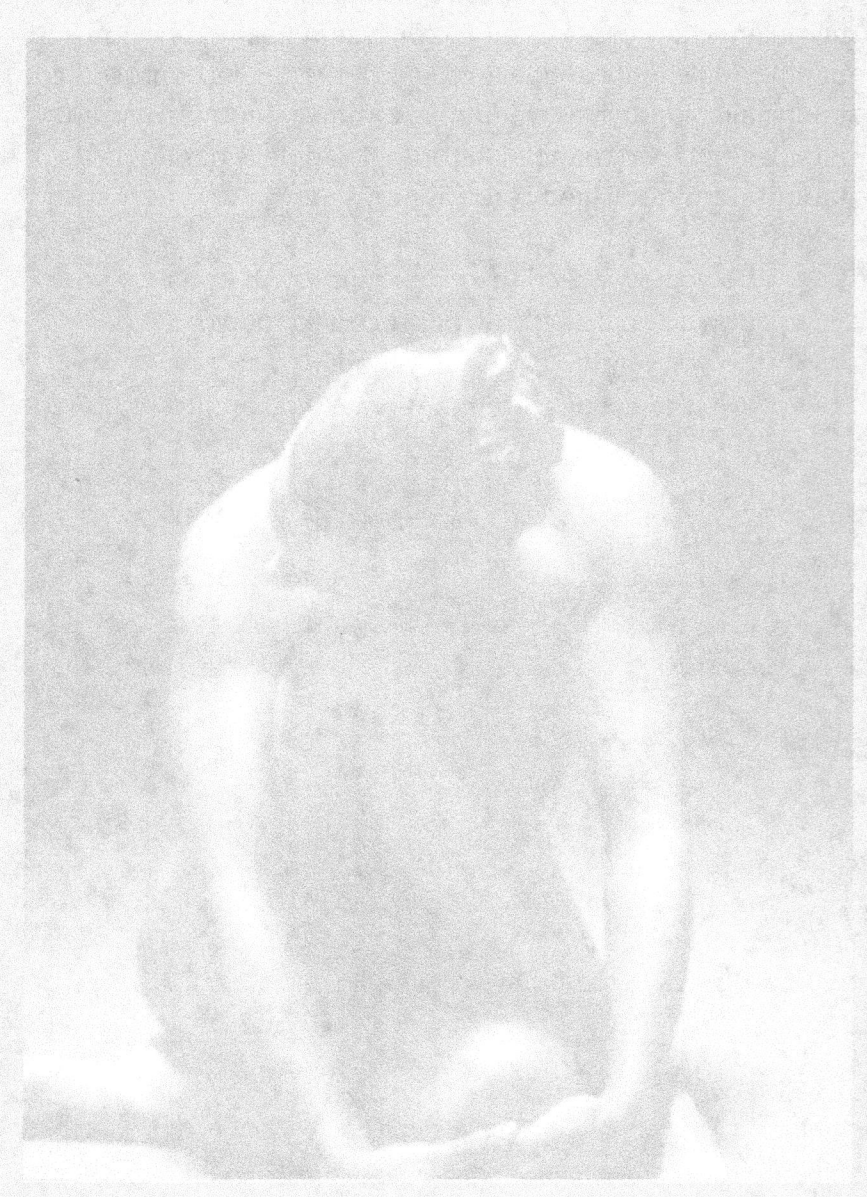

THE FOURTH SECRET:
LIFE'S OTHER PLEASURES

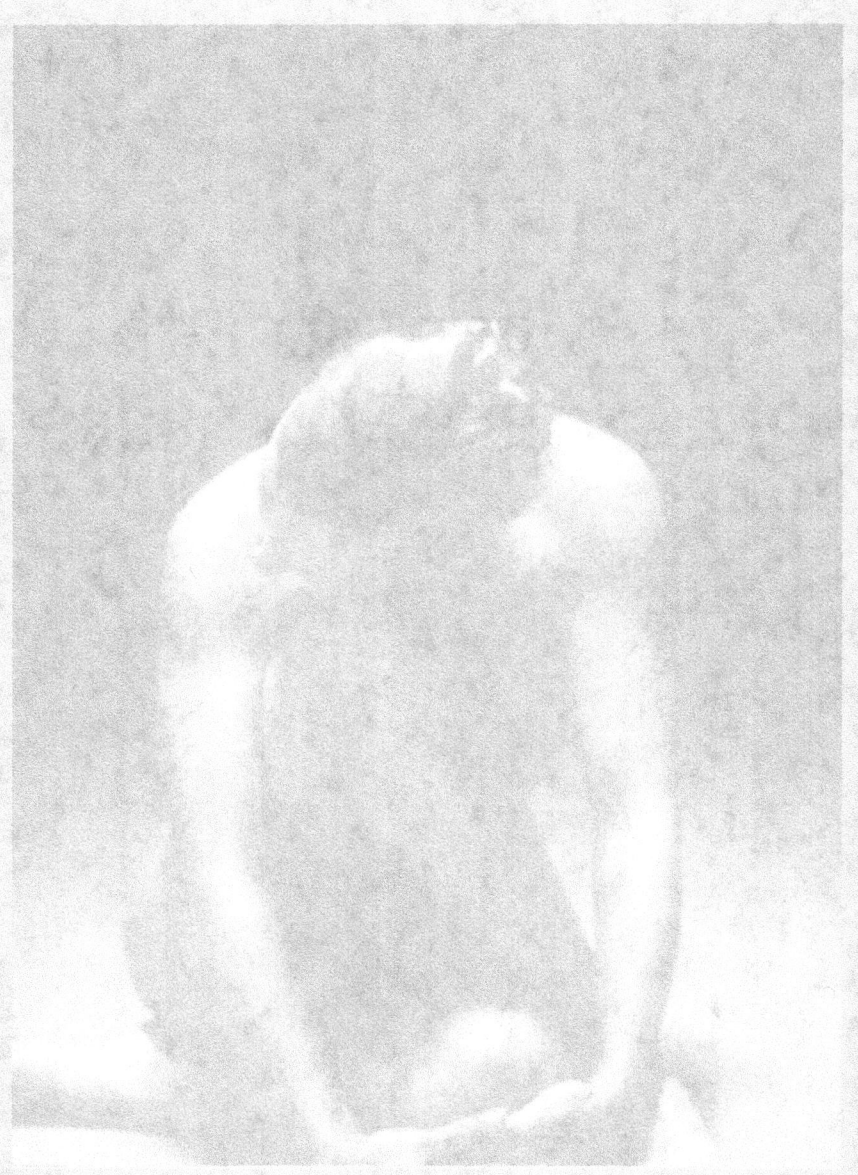

When I am in the throes of a binge, I lose my mind: I can see nothing in front of me. I can think of nothing wholesome or health-giving. I am gripped by obsession. I lose perspective of so many aspects of living that give me pleasure outside of food. For example, I love the beach, especially in the early morning, while the air is still cool and fresh, the beach is empty and quiet save for the squeals of the gulls mingled in with the rush of the tide on the sand. Few things delight me more than that.

Of course, I cannot be at the beach at a moment's notice. What about other pleasures? I love to curl up with an engrossing book and lose myself in the story. I love taking a refreshing shower and the cool feeling that I have stepping into clean clothes. I love freshly-washed bedsheets: My sleep is especially deep on new bedsheets. A very pleasurable activity is walking outdoors on a Sunday morning, before the rush of traffic, before the awakening crowd. I also love coffee. It may well be one of my favorite foods. I love getting up very early in the morning, before anyone in the household has arisen, and sitting quietly with my own cup of coffee that I don't have to share! Sounds selfish? It isn't. This is my quiet time.

What are your favorite things? Your other pleasures? List them here. Dwell on them. Explore them deeply.

- Favorite activity
- Favorite time of day
- Favorite time of year
- Favorite music

If money were no object, how would you design your life in such a way as to experience more pleasure? Allow yourself to dream – dreaming is free!

- What is your perfect day like?
- Would you quit your job?
- Would you contemplate an affair?

THE FIFTH SECRET: SELF-ESTEEM

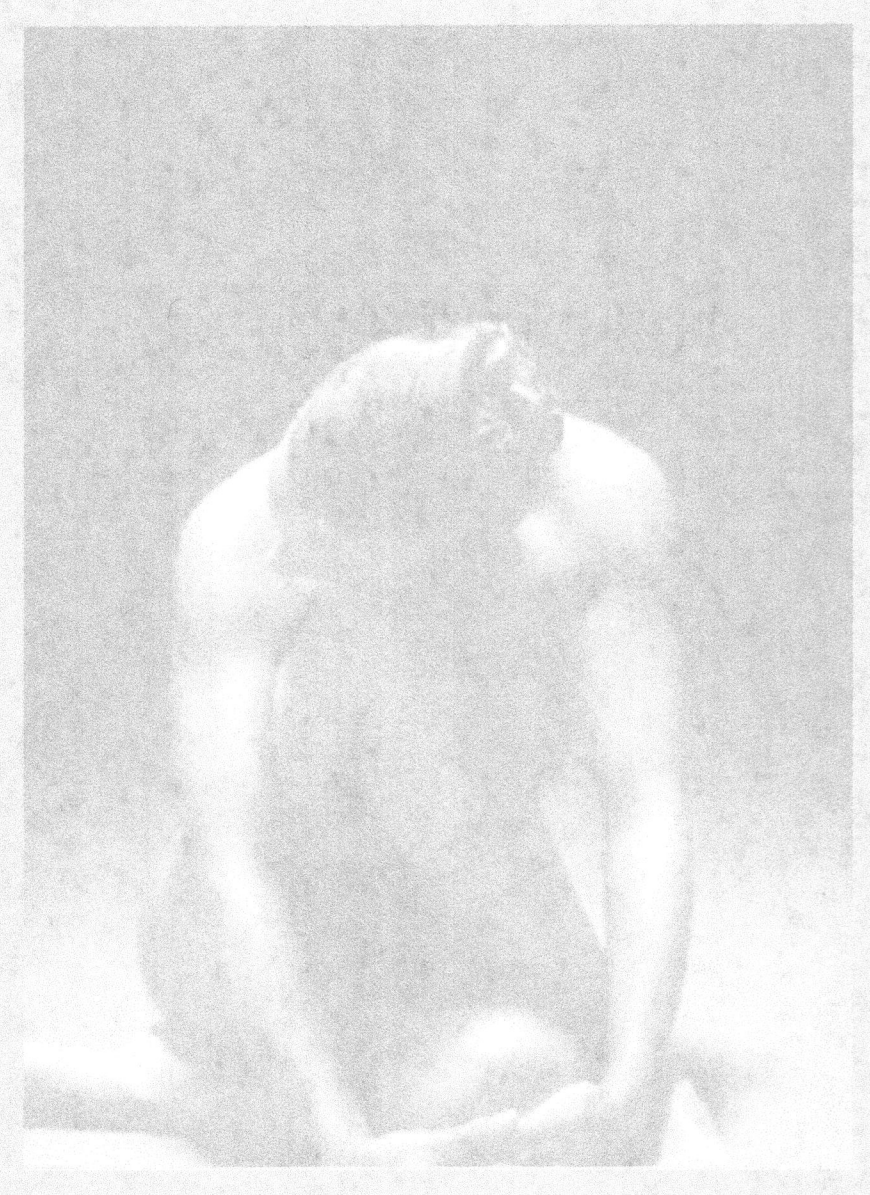

Self-esteem has nothing to do with conceit. It is a form of self love that transcends self-importance. On the contrary: self-esteem acknowledges a measure of humility. Self-esteem is a sense of confidence, a realization that you are strong enough, courageous enough, plucky enough to get it done. Get what done? The hard stuff. Do you cringe at the prospect of a big project, but do it anyway? Do you complain about the heavy assignment load your professor gave you, but plod through it anyway, and complete it well? That is self-esteem. You have to know yourself, trust your abilities, trust your commitment to the job, trust your word to have self-esteem.

Give an example – or several – of having accomplished a difficult task successfully?

- Completed a difficult project – describe it
- Completed an advanced degree
- Cared for a dying relative

How did you feel during the process?

- Exhausted
- Resentful
- Comfortable
- Successful/proud

Did the entire process go smoothly? If not, describe it here.

What was particularly difficult or onerous about the project?

What made you stick through it?

How did you feel when you were finished?

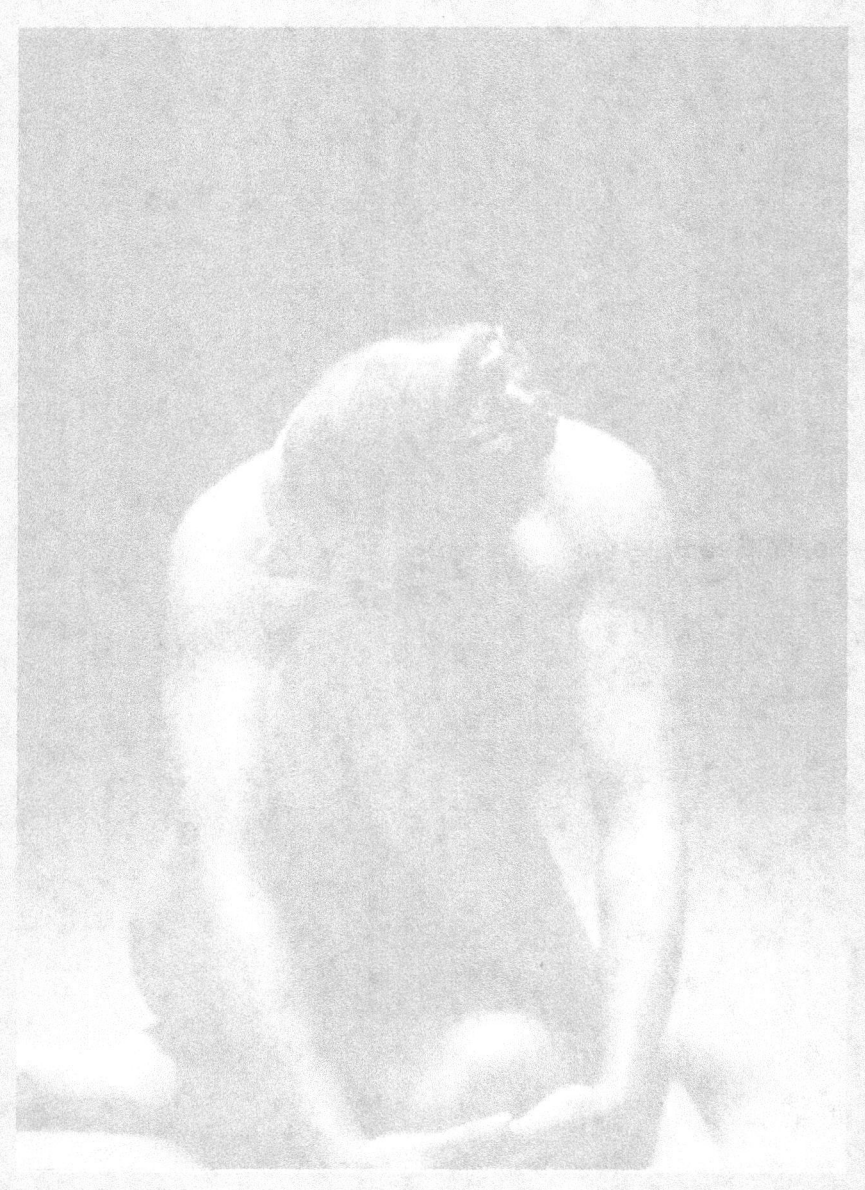

THE SIXTH SECRET: INTEGRITY

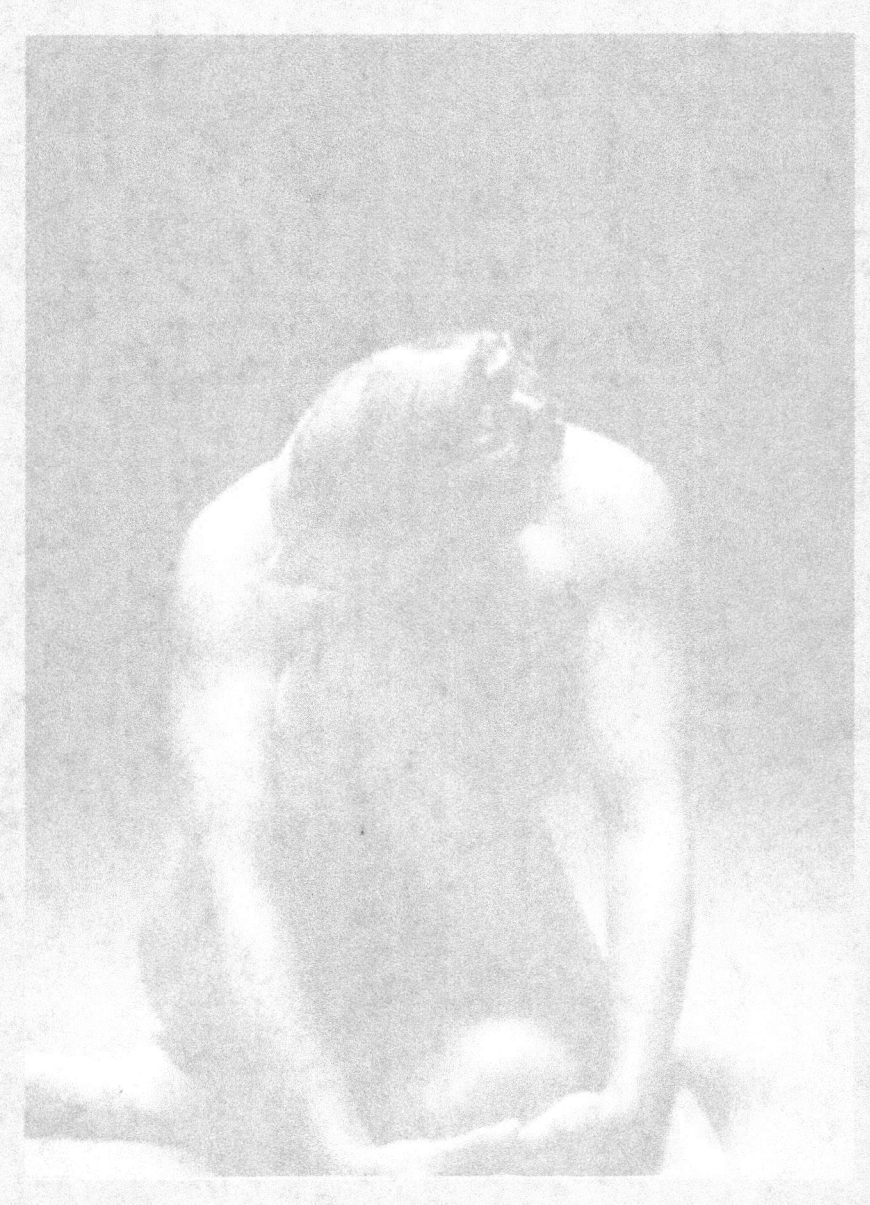

Integrity is a complicated concept, akin to honesty, but deeper. Integrity means whole, and whole in this sense means being holistic, being true to one's standards of right and wrong. In its simplest terms, it means keeping your word – to others as to yourself. If something does not feel right, trust your intuition, because its integrity may be "out" or missing. Something is askew, and your inner self can sense it. Just as you know when someone is lying to you, so you can sense when something does not feel right. This is true of your relationships, your job, your friends and most importantly, yourself.

- Are you living a life of your own making, or placating to others' expectations of you?
- Do you feel independent/dependent?
- Do you have self-confidence?

Allow yourself to go deeply; examine your soul. This is your book, your private domain.

- Are you a pleaser? Whom are you trying to please?
- Do you always tell it like it is? If not, why not?
- Do you sometimes lie?

Can you be trusted to keep your word at all times and in all matters?

- Do you shirk responsibility, or welcome it eagerly?
- Do you volunteer for extra projects at work?
- Do you take on extra-credit work in school?
- When you feel overwhelmed or annoyed by a project, do you abandon it?

Do you give of yourself – your time, your talents – without expectation of a reward?

Do you resent saying yes so often? Would you like to say no – but don't? Why?

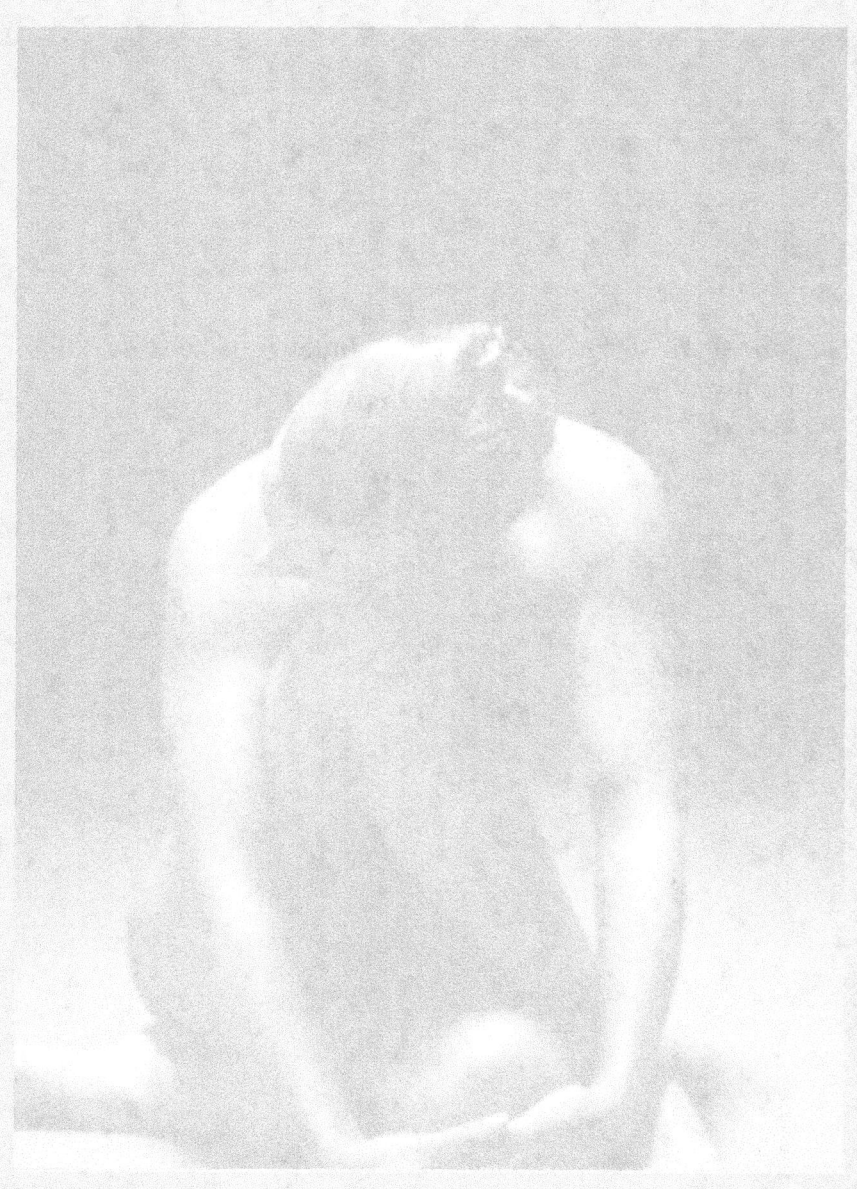

THE SEVENTH SECRET:
GRATITUDE

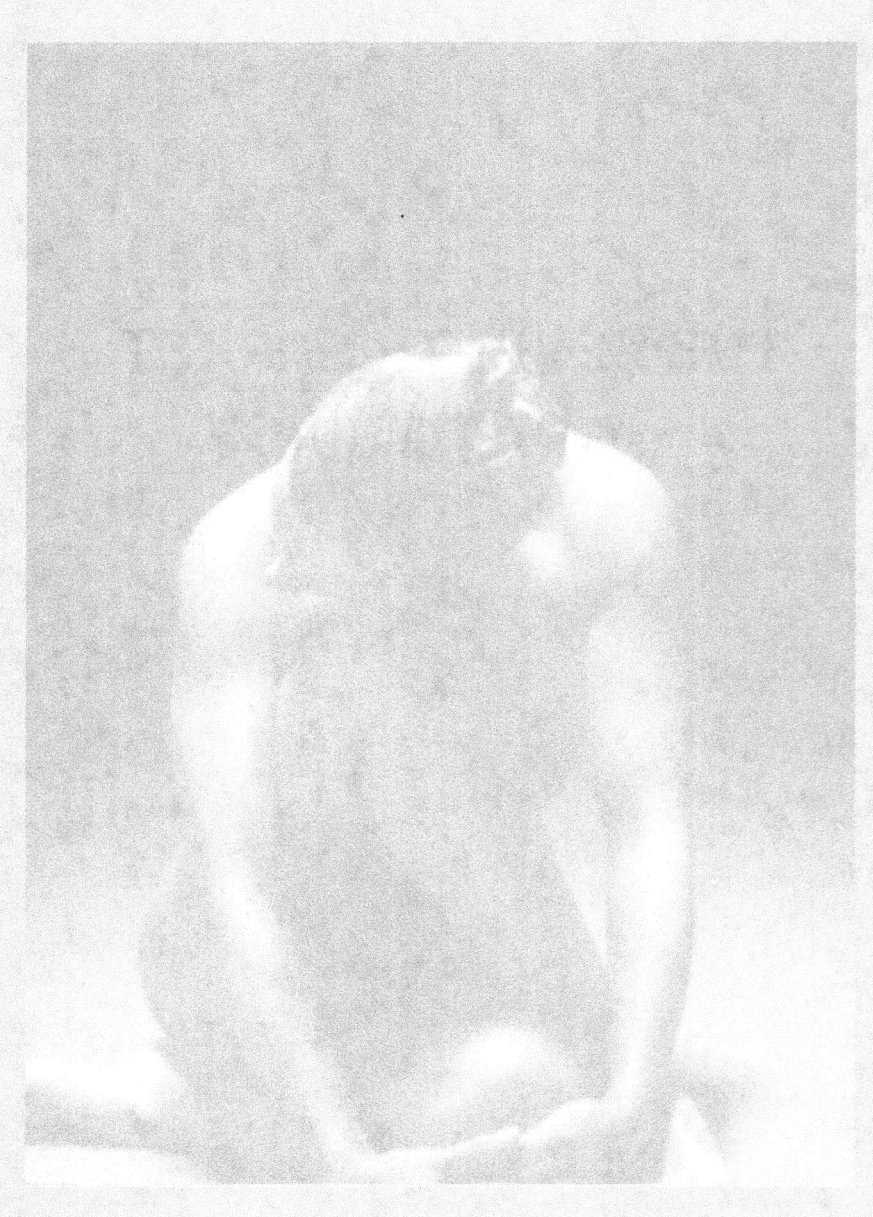

Just as life's other pleasures, so is gratitude prominently emblazoned in my heart. I live in Florida, my piece of heaven on earth. What percentage of the world's population is so lucky to live in paradise? I am grateful for every succulent, sunny day and cool, refreshing evening. I am even grateful for the winters in Florida that are so gentle and short-lived. I am grateful for my health and beauty. I can sing, and am grateful for my voice. I am grateful that I love fresh fruits and vegetables, and don't push them off my plate, but devour them hungrily. I am grateful for my intelligence and abilities, my financial savvy, my ability to enjoy complex reading material; indeed, I am grateful for my ability to read!

This is your journal, your own domain. Please give yourself free rein to list each and every thing, person or situation you are grateful for. Remember to list your difficulties as well, as those are the best teachers.

Most of all, I am grateful for the opportunity to write this book and offer it to you.

EPILOGUE

The best diet you will ever need is the one that sustains you in happiness and good health – physical and emotional. I sincerely hope I have been able to impart some concepts that will serve as beacons on your own journey. I wish you success, pleasure and good health!

Remember: It's not about the food – it's all about you!

Thank you for taking this journey with me!

www.ingramcontent.com/pod-product-compliance
Lightning Source LLC
Chambersburg PA
CBHW062119280526
45787CB00009B/1196